POSITIVE THINKING

*Transform your life with the
power of thinking positively!*

Alicia Wilkinson, MSW, LCSW

Positive Thinking

Positive Thinking	1
Disclaimer	5
Introduction	6
Are You An Optimist or Pessimist?	7
Optimistic People	8
Pessimistic People	9
Which One Are You?	10
How Can You Train Your Mind to Think Positively?	11
Understanding Negativity	12
Take Control of Your Thoughts	12
Interrupt the Negative	13
Redirect and Reframe	13
Transform Your Health Through Positive Thinking	15
Daily Affirmations	16
Connections and Community	17
Contribute as Much as you Consume	17
Do What You Love	18
Why Is It Important to Think Positive	19
Inner Beauty Becomes Outer Beauty	20
Opportunities Replace Problems	20
Boost of Self-Esteem and Motivation	21
Better Health and Wellness	21
Enriched Relationships	21
Success	22
Positivity Attracts More Positivity	22

Do You Have a Positive Self Image? 23
Do You Have a Solid Foundation of Self-Worth? 24
Do You Feel Those Around You Define Who You Are? 24
Do You Give Power to Self-Criticism and Self-Judgment? 25
Are You Codependent? 25
Do You Love You? 26

A Positive Attitude at Work Can Boost Your Success 27
What To Do – and What Not To Do 28
Office Gossip is a No-Go 28
Be a Team Player 28
Don't Be A Serial Complainer 28
Keep Your Potty Mouth Shut 29
Advantages of a Positive Attitude at Work 29
You'll Be a Role Model 29
Health and Wellness 29
Lead Roles 29
Promotion, Promotion, Promotion! 30

Positive Thinking is Great, Positive 'Action' is Better! 31
Emotion First, Then Behavior 32
Professional Example 32
Personal Example 32
Social Example 33
Behavior First, Then Emotion 33
Professional Example 33
Personal Example 33
Social Example 34
Completing the Circle of Self-motivation 34

Tips to Overcome Negative Thoughts 35
Eggs, Bacon and Positivity! 36
Give Negative Surroundings the Boot! 36
Word Purge! 37
Q and A Time! 37
Search and Rescue! 38

Reduce Stress by Reducing Negative Self-Talk 39
Permit Imperfections 40
Choose Your Words 41
Avoid Assumptions 41
Jot It Down 41
Promote a Positive Self-Image 42

Benefits of Positive Thinking 43
More Effective Coping Skills 44
A Healthier, Longer Life 44
Appreciate the Good Things 44
Success 45

Acknowledgments 47

Disclaimer

We hope you enjoy reading this publication, however we do suggest you read our disclaimer. All the material written in this document is provided for informational purposes only and is general in nature.

Every person is a unique individual and what has worked for some or even many may not work for you. Any information perceived as advice by must be considered in light of your own particular set of circumstances.

The author or person sharing this information does not assume any responsibility for the accuracy or outcome of your use of the content.

Every attempt has been made to provide well researched and up to date content at the time of writing. Now all the legalities have been taken care of, please enjoy the content.

Introduction

At times it feels as if you are drowning. No shore insight, with life's obstacles weighing you down. Do you feel God will have to move mountains just so you can catch a breath of air?

One of the biggest, if not *the* biggest, determinants of happiness and success is a person's attitude and expectation. That is, are they a positive thinking person, confident in their own ability?

Do they have an expectation that life will deliver good things to them, even in those times when their ability might be lacking?

So many people have turned their lives around by changing their attitude to themselves, to others and life in general. Like anything that delivers worthwhile results, real effort is required.

This effort is mostly emotional rather than physical, although some of the very real benefits are huge improvements in health, longevity and quality of life. The point is, anyone can do it, and benefit from it, if they put in the action required.

Positive thinking is one of those areas where it gets easier as it goes on. Little actions yield small successes, but these multiply, to a state where they then seem to occur constantly, without noticeable effort.

This book has the potential to unlock potential in you that may be being held back by long-held fears and behaviors. It provides understanding of why and how positive thinking works to improve life's outcomes, and very practical and easy-to follow steps to help overcome negativity and embrace a positive attitude.

Are You An Optimist or Pessimist?

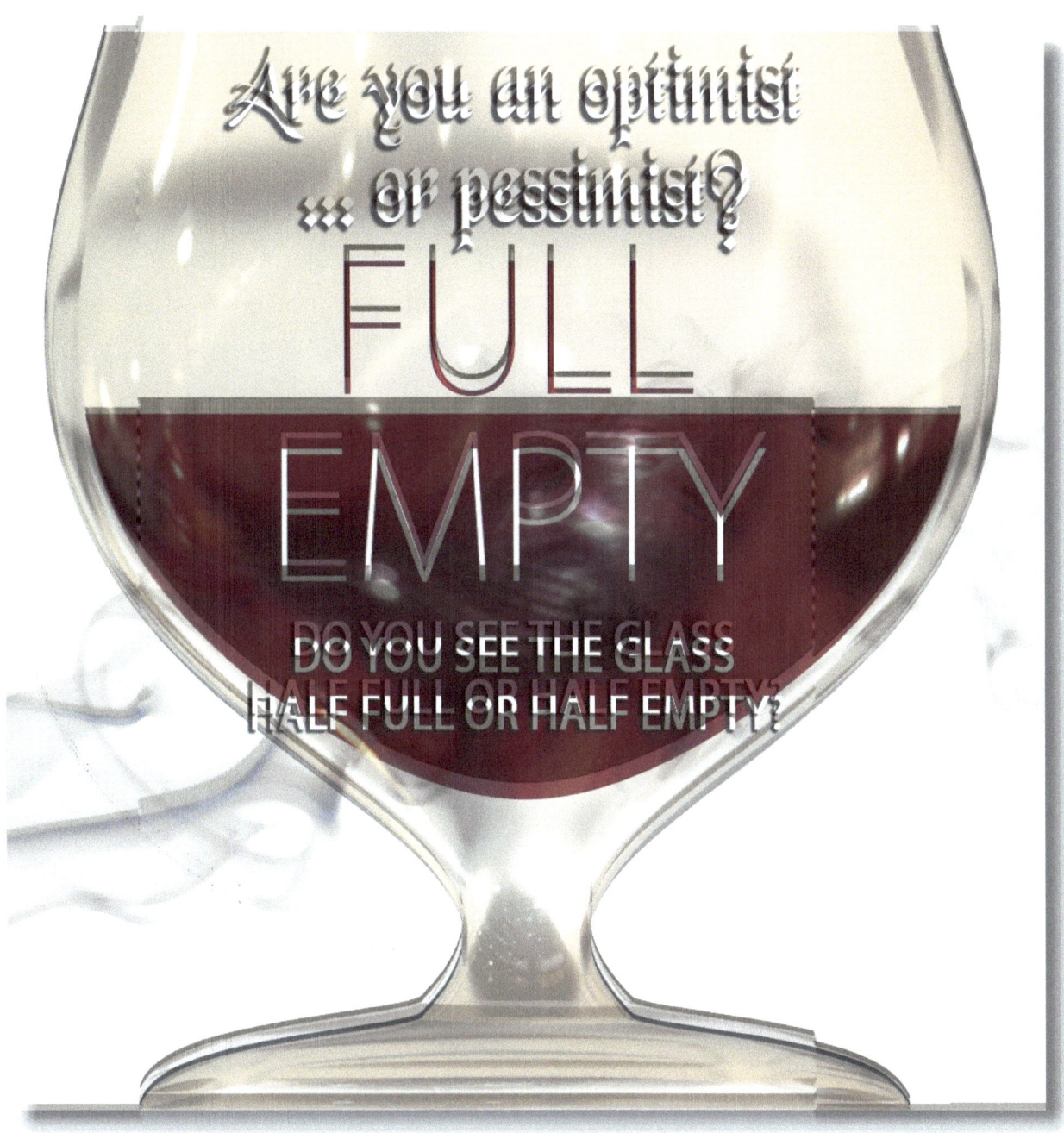

There is an excellent quote that sums up the difference between optimism and pessimism, and that's the one by Winston Churchill.

"A pessimist sees the difficulty in every opportunity; an optimist sees the opportunity in every difficulty."

Optimism and pessimism are a combination of attitude, perception and overall approach to life's circumstances.

Do you believe you are an optimist or pessimist? Can you be both? Is one better than the other? The general opinion is that optimism is better because optimistic people seem to be happier no matter what comes their way.

However, one could also argue that pessimism has some perks too. Let's take a look at each trait in more detail.

Optimistic People

The glass is always half-full for these people. No matter the situation, they will always find something good. Problems aren't even really problems in a sense, they just sort of think of "problems" as obstacles they have to overcome or a stepping stone to something greater.

Their attitude shines through to those around them and they are easy to be around. In fact, people are more likely to be attracted to an optimistic personality *because* of their happiness and demeanor.

Self-confidence is also a striking trait optimistic people portray. Instead of dodging problems, they tend to go head-on and face whatever is coming their way. They also seem to rely on faith and perseverance in difficult situations.

Even if they've been thrown a curveball, they will find the positive. Optimistic people focus more on solutions than the problem itself. Slow to be disappointed, they will reframe opposition and look at it as a lesson learned.

Here's an example: 'Optimistic Olivia' has just applied for a position within her place of current employment offering a substantial raise and a fancy title. She might even score a parking space closer to the building entrance!

She's got all her ducks in a row, and has practiced potential interview questions in front of the mirror. She's confident when she walks into the interview, and afterwards feels good about how it went.

When she gets the news that the position went to another person in her office, with lesser qualifications, she doesn't let it upset her. Instead, 'Optimistic Olivia' shifts her thoughts and disappointment and believes there is something even better waiting for her.

In the meantime, she still goes above and beyond at work and keeps a positive attitude towards everyone, even the person who beat her out of the position.

Pessimistic People

These are the 'glass is always half-empty' kind of folks, and it's probably contaminated water anyway. The future is going to be a disappointment, so why even look forward to it?

They find it hard to get their hopes up about something because it's never going to turn out in their favor, so they just prepare themselves for the worst. That way, it's not so devastating.

Pessimistic people seem to display regret and use words expressing finality, like "all", "nothing", "everything", and "always" to describe their situations. They have an uncanny ability to find fault wherever they look and it's usually someone else's fault for their unhappiness.

Living in self-pity is a trait of theirs and they have a tendency to give up easily. Problems can easily be seen as catastrophic events and they will frequently display hateful and discouraging behavior to those around them, especially optimistic people. It's almost as if they find a secret joy in destroying happiness; theirs and others.

Here's an example: 'Pessimistic Patty' is applying for the same job as 'Optimistic Olivia'. She doesn't think she will get it because she feels her coworkers don't like her. She doesn't prepare for the interview (because she won't get it anyway) and this in turn makes her very nervous and self-conscious.

Low and behold she gets the job, but she doesn't find any joy in hearing the news. Instead, she believes her coworkers are going to *really* hate her even worse and now she will have much more responsibility.

'Pessimistic Patty's' focus turns to concern. What if she's fired when they realize she can't handle the new job duties? She starts to regret even applying.

Which One Are You?

Do you find yourself thinking more negatively or positively? If you can turn any situation around and find the good, you're probably an optimistic person. Likewise, if anything and everything has a negative connotation, you might just be pessimistic.

The good news is both optimism and pessimism are choices we make. Which one do you think you are right now? Is it the one you would like to be?

How Can You Train Your Mind to Think Positively?

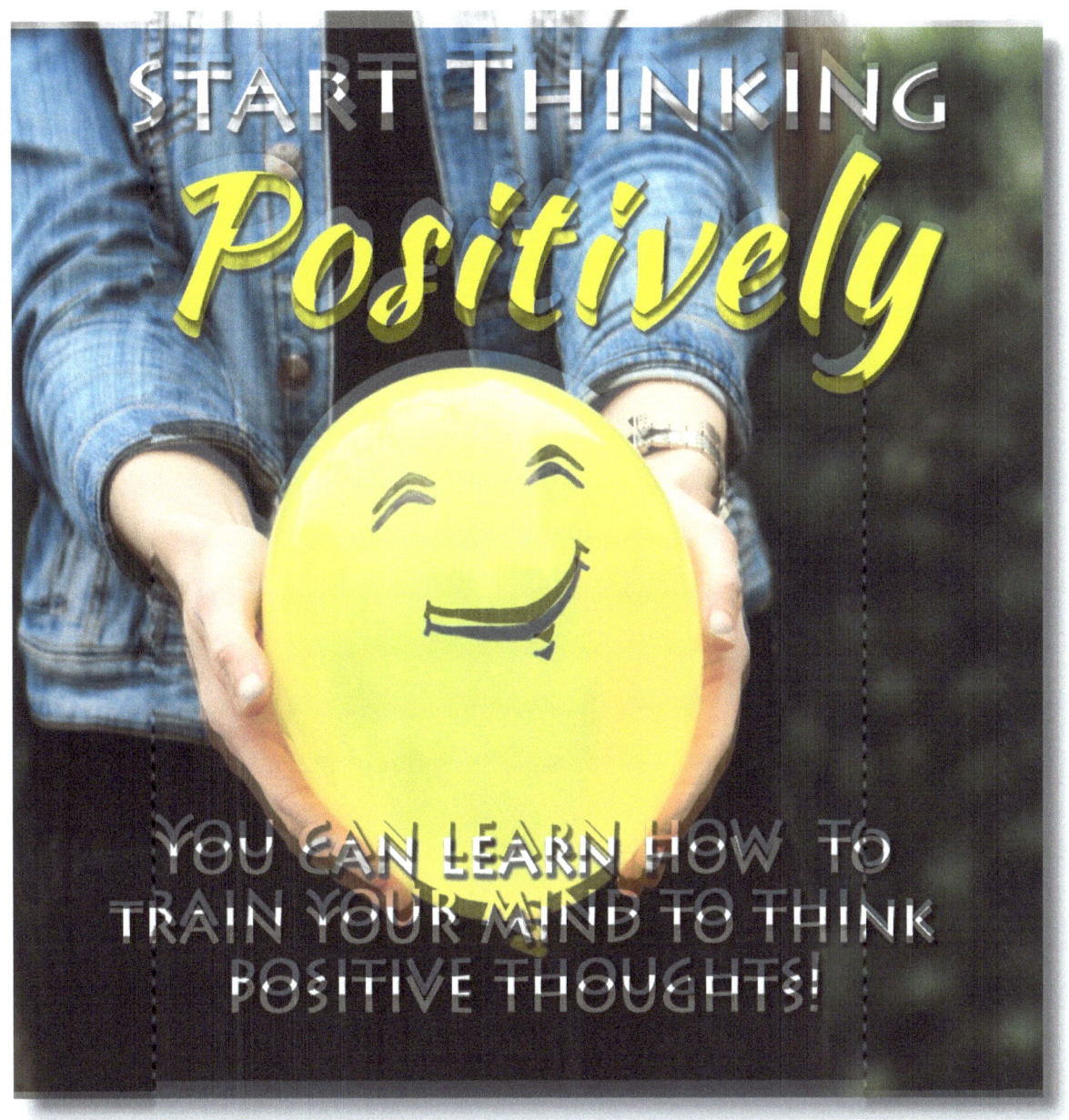

The brain is a powerful tool. Every life experience marks a notch in our brain, with the ultimate goal of survival. Being happy and thinking positively aren't things that come naturally to many of us, especially if we've allowed life and external events to determine our mood and attitude.

The good news is you can train your mind to find that ray of sunshine, the light at the end of the tunnel, the good in any situation, *if* you give it the proper tools and apply them. If you find yourself thinking more on the negative side, keep reading.

We will explore several ways for you to get control over your mind and think positively!

Understanding Negativity

First, we need to fully understand where all the negativity is coming from before we can stop it. Our minds take every situation and go into survival mode. The brain recognizes the difficulty in any given situation and provides you with the *easiest* and *quickest* way to get out of it.

Then it locks in these painful memories and difficult situations and refers to them in times of stress, giving us a reference point on how to deal with what's happening now.

It's automatic. It's a pattern. This is unconscious behavior, and it served our primitive ancestors well, keeping them safe from the many harms that availed them. And we *allow* it, because escape or avoidance is easier than going head-on into difficult times and persevering with positivity.

We are assigning more power to the negative than positive. The recurring negative thoughts become second nature and it affects every aspect of our lives. It's time to break the cycle and learn how to think positively!

Take Control of Your Thoughts

Easier said than done, right? Sometimes our thoughts just run rampant and we don't even realize it. Before you know it you're in a foul mood simply because you've let a negative thought sequence take over your entire mood. Acknowledge your thoughts.

- What are you thinking about right now?
- Are your thoughts causing you distress or supporting a happy disposition?

Pay attention to how your body is reacting to your thoughts. Be aware of how you are breathing, how your body feels and reacts to any given circumstance.

You have the power to think about whatever you want. You have the ultimate say in where your mind goes and what you choose to focus on, be it good or bad. But first you have to acknowledge and take control.

However, this does require some degree of conscious, *mindful* effort. As explained, our subconscious is dedicated to our survival. Stepping above that, to improving ourselves, and our attitude and perspective, requires engaging our conscious, thinking, rational mind.

Interrupt the Negative

When you pay attention to what's on your mind, make a determination:

*Is this thought supporting my goals and the overall attitude I want,
or is this thought hindering me?*

If your thought is negative and you don't want it to control your mind, interrupt it. It takes a bit of practice, but you'll get it. In the beginning you'll find your mind wandering back to the negativity, but gently and persistently interrupt that thought.

Redirect and Reframe

Now that you've taken the negative thought and isolated it, it's time to redirect and reframe. Turn this thought into something positive, no matter how difficult or mundane it may seem. From the simplest to the most complex, turn it around and force your mind to think about something positive in direct relation to this thought.

For instance, you're in line at the grocery store waiting for your turn to check out. Your mind starts wandering because you're idle. You start thinking about a fight you had with your partner last night, and it didn't end well. Your body responds and starts to tense up and your pulse increase.

Now you are feeling upset and inpatient, and without realizing it you snap at the lady working the register because she's not moving fast enough.

You've given so much power to the negative thought! It has complete control and swallowed up any chance you had at being happy today. Now you feel defeated and like your entire day will be downhill from here on out.

Now try the same scenario this way:

- Acknowledge the thought: *Yes, there was an argument and I don't like how it ended.*
- Interrupt: *Stop! I'm not going to allow this negativity to have power over my day.*
- Redirect/Reframe: *I can't fix this right now, but I'll be more compassionate when I get home and try to listen better. We will have a great night!*

You can do this with virtually any negative situation and find the good. Feeling the anger is easy. Put more effort into ways to fix the situation thus removing the power from negativity and replacing it with positivity.

Again, it takes some practice but it will soon become second nature and you'll be able to replace negativity with positivity without even trying!

Transform Your Health Through Positive Thinking

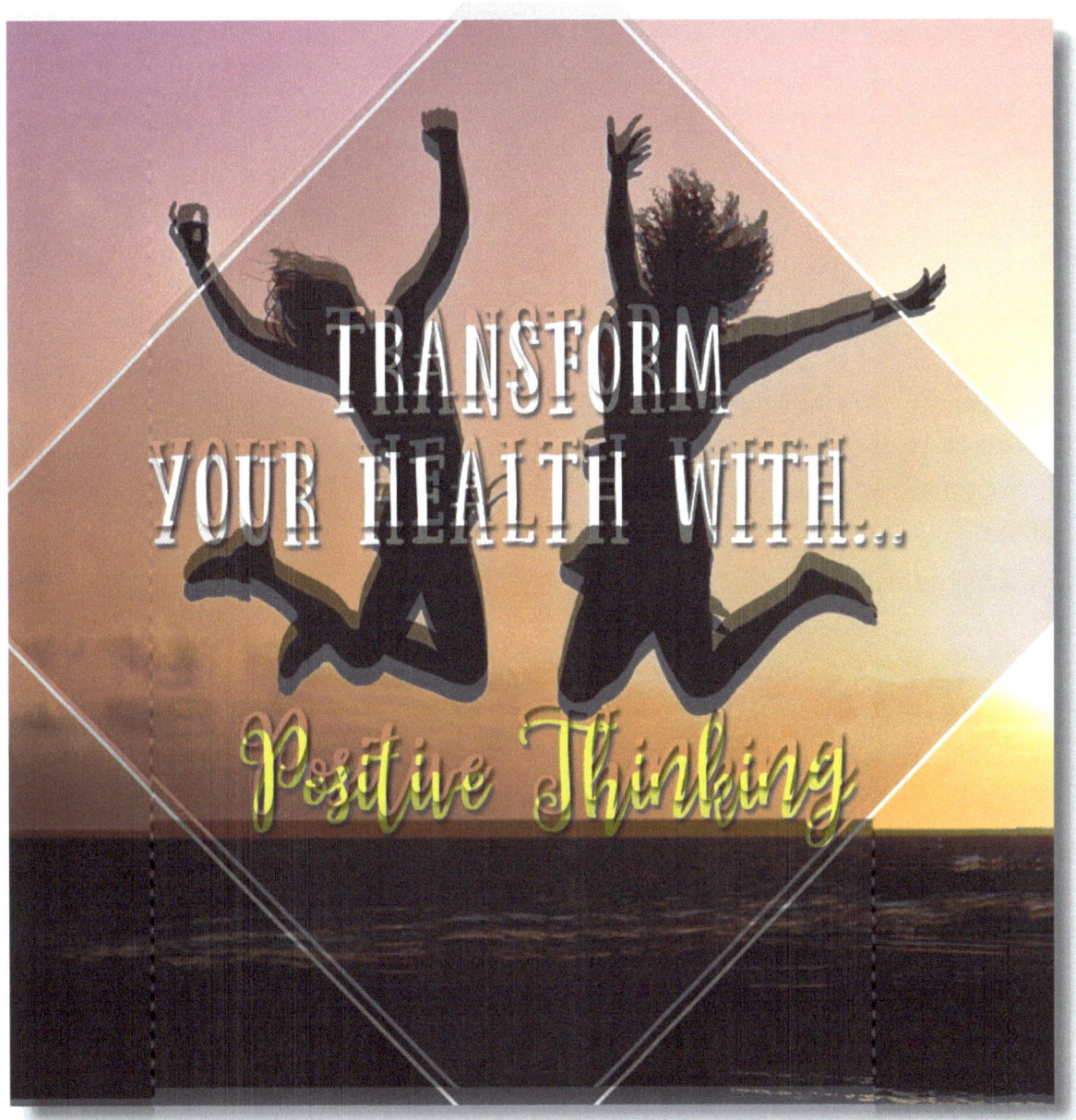

Everyone is hopping on the train for health and wellness, it seems, and that has to be a good thing. People are jumping through hoops to try this diet or another, working out at the gym like crazy until they *feel* better.

Spending money on personal trainers and nutrition specialists to finally hit a high point in life they so desperately crave.

It's astounding how many folks have yet to learn how important positive thinking is to their overall health and wellness. Physical, mental and spiritual health begins on the inside. You can actually transform your health through positive thinking!

That's not to say exercise and a proper diet aren't part of the process, but when you feel better *inside*, you are more apt to work on the *outside*. The decisions you make for your health will become much easier and second nature when you are happy and creating a chock-full existence for yourself and those around you.

When you are looking forward with positive anticipation to your end-goal, you will find yourself 'doing what needs to done', with less effort. Compare this to the begrudging effort required otherwise.

Daily Affirmations

Quite possibly the easiest and least used method to start your day with joy and positivity, daily affirmations pave the way for success, happiness and insight. You could do anything from hand-written notes stuck on your bathroom mirror, fridge and coffee maker to utilizing your smart phone for reminders throughout the day.

There are countless ways to get in your daily affirmations. The challenge is in giving them power. It's not enough just to see them. Empower these power tools by stating them out loud, with conviction and an open mind.

Need examples of how to encourage your best self?

- *Today is going to be fantastic because I won't let anything get in the way of my positivity.*
- *I have the power to control my actions and reactions; I will use it wisely.*
- *This is the beginning of a great day; I can't wait to see how well I handle it!*
- *I am strong, beautiful, courageous and smart; I am the key to my own happiness!*

When you *feel good*, you *react good*. Don't let your inner self take a hit because you aren't prepared for the day. Arm yourself with positivity first thing in the morning and all through the day. Give yourself the tools necessary to create a positive environment.

Connections and Community

Here's a doozy. Technology has made so many advances we can essentially live in a virtual world without human contact. We can work from home, have friends and family interact with our social media posts, and even have meals delivered right to our doorstep.

It's entirely possible to live as a complete shut-in without human interaction. But we *need* people. Humans are social creatures. Our brains crave conversational stimulation and interaction. Our emotions need close connections and community to fully develop and feel whole.

Need some ideas on how to develop positive, healthy connections?

- Join a book club or craft group
- Attend church and participate in small groups sessions
- Visit friends and family, show interest in their lives

When you develop strong connections within your community it creates a feeling of self-confidence and inner growth. You are more equipped to deal with the challenges of day-to-day life when you've got the proper tools and know-how. Engaging in social interaction initiates a positive outlook for a multitude of life's puzzling moments.

Contribute as Much as you Consume

Volunteer, donate and give back. If you find yourself wishing you had more in life, give more. It doesn't have to be money either. Offer your time to a homeless shelter, an animal shelter, a food bank, a local hospital, or any number of places looking for volunteers. Random acts of kindness are so incredibly fulfilling.

Giving *feels* good. Feeling productive and knowing you are part of the solution instead of ignoring the problem goes a long way in nurturing mental and spiritual health. When you are feeling negative, try 'paying it forward'. You can physically feel your negativity slipping away and in its place an abundance of positivity takes over.

Venture Outdoors

A bit of fresh air is good for the soul. Take a morning or afternoon walk. Go on a hiking adventure. Explore your city or town on foot, taking time to meet new people and visit local shops. Your lungs will thank you, and so will your level of joy and positivity.

Do What You Love

Not everyone is afforded the opportunity to be in love with their job. If that's your case, take time to do something you enjoy. We mark things down in our calendars and schedule just about everything. Why not add in there an allotted time for you to have fun?

Take a pottery class or join in on a yoga class. What's your pleasure? Crafts? Photography? Cooking? Do it. Make it happen. And watch your positivity soar! When you are happy, prepared and looking forward to the day, your stress level decreases which helps with blood pressure, cardiovascular health, anxiety, depression and overall well-being.
You are more likely to make better decisions when you are less stressed and can think objectively. Journal your progress and pay attention to how much better your health is after you've employed positive thinking strategies. You'll be astounded at the difference it makes!

Why Is It Important to Think Positive

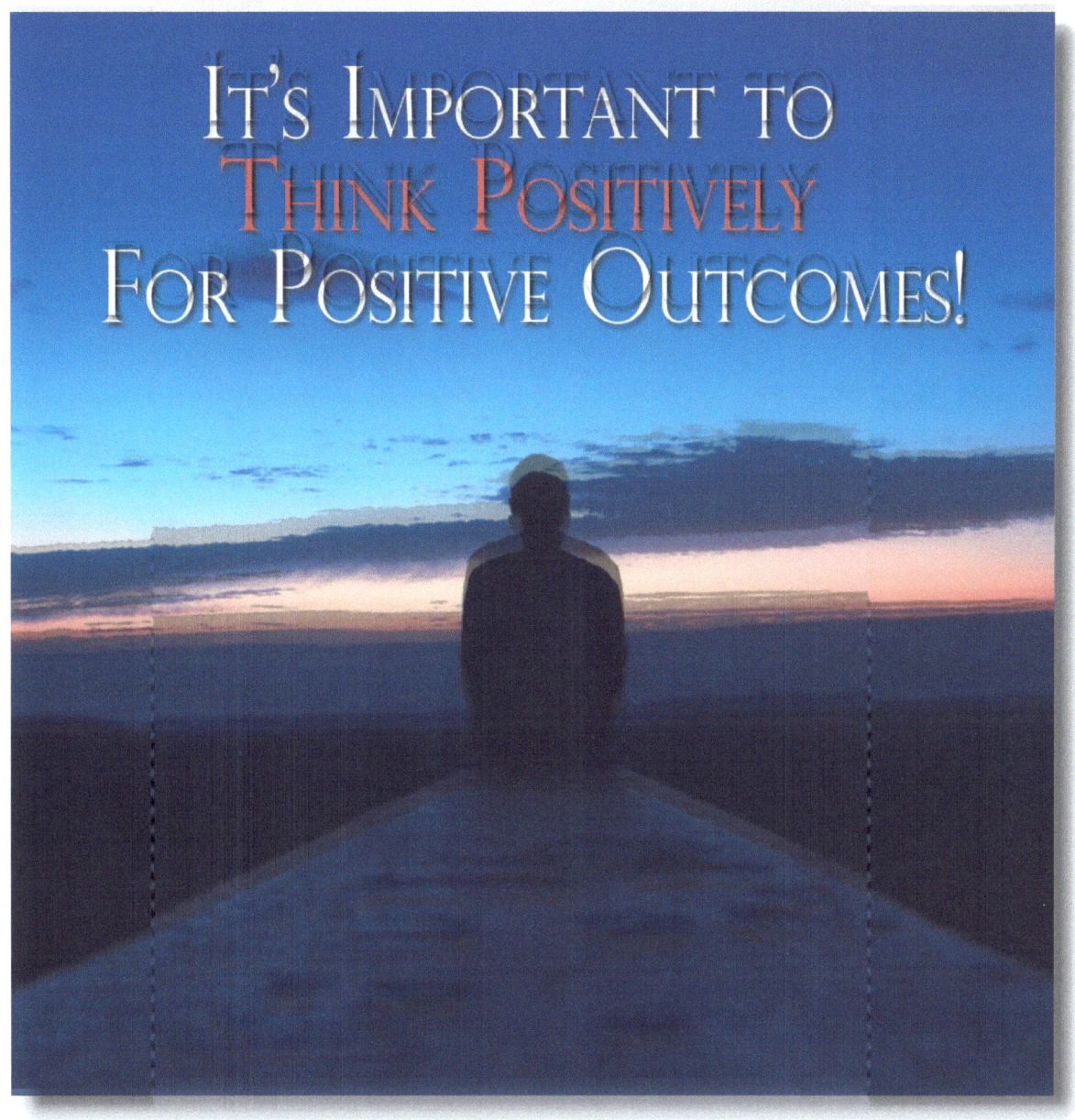

Thinking positive isn't just about being able to look at the glass half full. There are many facets of life a positive thought process can affect. Surely you can name off one or two pretty negative people you've encountered in day-to-day life. Do a quick assessment on their overall achievements, growth, social circle and health:

Now look at some of the positive people you know. When you do the same assessment it should be more than clear who has the healthier, happier and more abundant life. Let's break down a few of the reasons why it's important to think positively.

Inner Beauty Becomes Outer Beauty

People who think positive feel good about themselves on the inside. This inner beauty transforms into an outer beauty that simply cannot be measured. We all have flaws, but a positive thinker doesn't perseverate on the negative.

There are things each and every one of us can say we need to work on physically, but that positive attitude on a person shines and allows us to be more aware of the beauty in spite of the blemishes. As others take notice, it's even more encouraging and we subconsciously radiate more of the same.

Opportunities Replace Problems

One of the best attributes of a positive thinker is the ability to see opportunities whereas a negative thinker sees problems. Negative people get caught up in the problem itself and believe there is no way out, or if there is a way out they still aren't satisfied with the outcome.

A person reframing situations in a positive manner will see any obstacle as an opportunity.

Lost a job? *There's something better right around the corner, I'm sure of it. I'll just touch up the ol' resume and give this a go!*
Kid giving you major attitude? *He's probably going through something he doesn't want to talk about; I'll plan a fun day for us to spend together, maybe he will open up. I want him to know I'm here for him.*

In both of the above examples, it is easy to see how negative perceptions and actions would lead to far less wanted outcomes.

Boost of Self-Esteem and Motivation

Angry, unsatisfied, negative people like to blame everyone but themselves for their unhappiness. A positive thinker gets a jolt of self-esteem and motivation because they praise themselves for a job well done.

Instead of wallowing in self-deprecation, the positive thinker has created the motivation to keep moving and get that happy high all over again. It feels good to be productive. To know you've gotten something accomplished.

Better Health and Wellness

Happy people live healthier lives. The placebo effect proves this theory. A positive attitude goes a long way here. Positive thinkers respond better to medical treatment. They also make better decisions about health and wellness in general.

Have you ever gone to a spin class where the instructor was a complete sourpuss? No way! They are joyful and motivating and have an abundant supply of positive energy!

Enriched Relationships

Personal and professional alike, relationships become easier and more fulfilling. Humans are social creatures by nature. We crave interaction with others and a positive thinker has the ability to grow and maintain binding relationships with one another.

A key component to healthy relationships is communication.

Instead of immediately placing blame on another person, like a negative thinker might do, a positive thinker can effectively convey their own feelings without attacking the other person.

It does wonders for personal relationships like marriages and with other loved ones, as well as when encountering unfavorable personalities in the workplace.

Success

Think about anyone you know who has success in their career. Usually a miserable old coot won't find much success in any field because they are too busy lingering on everything that *has* and *could* go wrong. They don't really like to take chances, because in their mind they have already set up for failure.

A positive thinker will try to achieve the impossible. If they meet resistance or defeat, they adjust their plan and continue to move forward. They don't focus on the loss, but on the potential growth and how to get there.

They take the attitude that 'those who think it can't be done shouldn't get in the way of those who are doing it'. Positive thinkers aren't ones to easily give up!

Positivity Attracts More Positivity

If you portray a positive attitude, you are more likely to draw in those around you with the same mindset. Birds of a feather, right? Good, positive vibes sent out into the universe are returned with more good and positive vibes.

If you want more positive people in your life, be a positive person. They will flock to you!

It's so important to live a life with a positive attitude. Thinking positive runs full circle. It establishes a life of cheerfulness and perseverance. You feel better inside and out, become more mindful and accomplished, and create satisfying and lasting relationships.

There is simply nothing negative to report about a positive existence.

Do You Have a Positive Self Image?

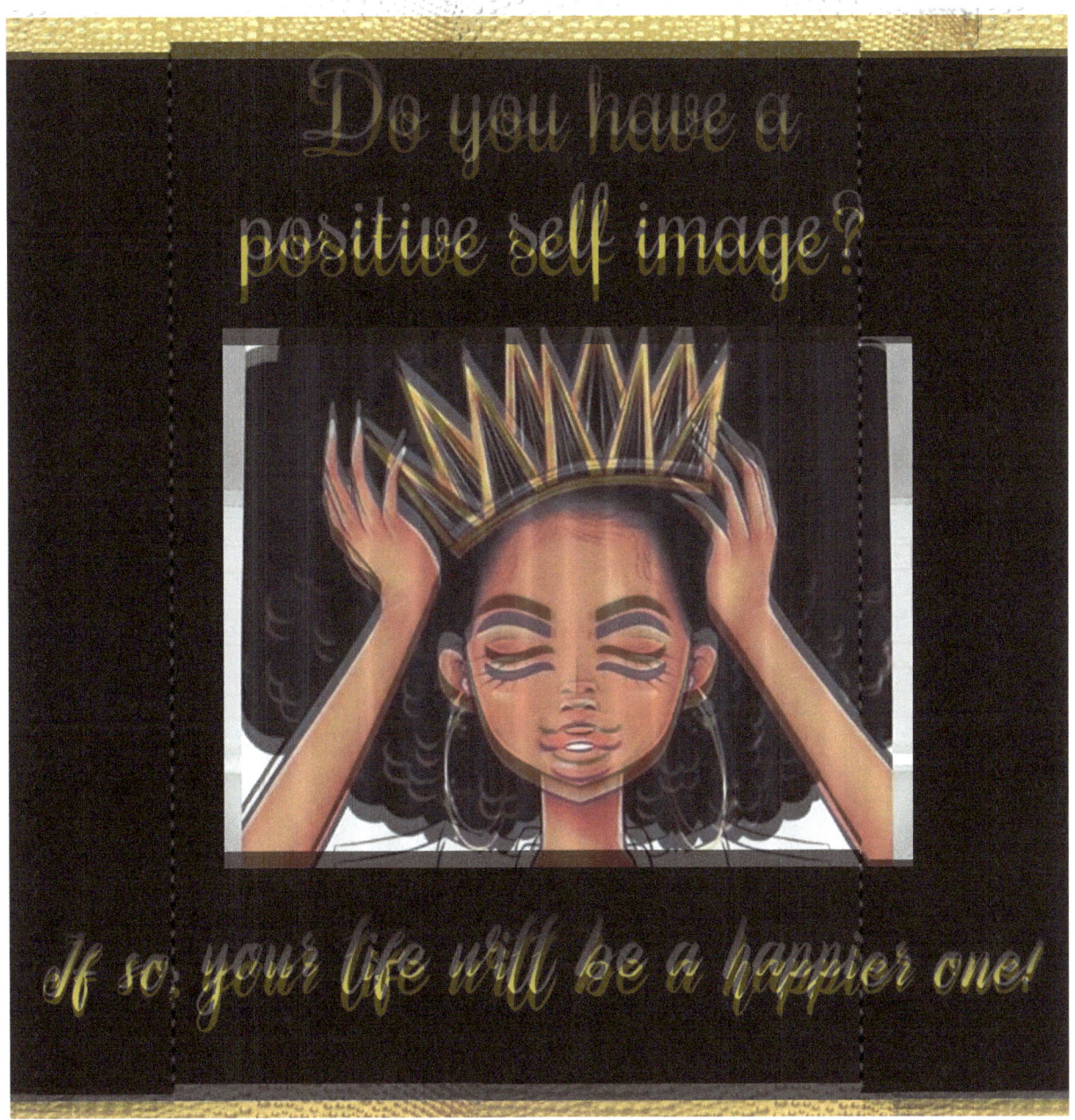

There's a constant battle in each of us with the opposing forces of positive and negative. How we *feel* about ourselves, inside and out, is what creates our self-image. More so, it's our *perception* of our own reality we have nurtured and cultivated over our entire lives to this point.

And it's constantly changing and evolving with time. Our self-image is the ultimate tour guide of our lives, and determines how we interact socially, emotionally and spiritually with any given circumstance or situation that arises.

Do you have a positive self-image? Below are a few key factors of those with a positive self-image and how they see themselves.

Do You Have a Solid Foundation of Self-Worth?

People with a positive self-image believe in themselves. They feel they are worthy of this life they have created and are happily living in it. Psychologists believe self-worth and self-image begin developing at a very young age.

Children who experienced play time in social groups and sports learned how to interact with others and developed a higher degree of social skills. They were able to accept the loss of a game or an argument with a buddy and move forward without much ado.

This paved the way for a high sense of self-worth, as well as physical and mental confidence as an adult. Alternately, children with underdeveloped social skills, or those who experienced childhood trauma, had a lesser opinion of themselves thus feeling more insecure and less confident as adults.

This affects all aspects of their lives, as it heavily impacts decision-making, which is a pillar of happiness and achievement.

Do You Feel Those Around You Define Who You Are?

If you are waiting for the approval of the world, your self-image might not be as positive as it could be. Those with a positive self-image don't typically seek the approval of others.

They do what they do for their own achievement and personal gain, not for the sole purpose of acknowledgement or approval of others. If they want to improve their lives, they do it. People with a positive self-image aren't indignant when they do a task and don't receive praise.

In fact, if you have a positive self-image you are more likely to be a trend-setter than a follower. Sure, praise is good and dandy, but it's just a side benefit in the grand scheme of things.

Do You Give Power to Self-Criticism and Self-Judgment?

People who have a positive self-image are confident in their own abilities, and just as importantly, more likely to perceive setbacks as feedback rather than failure.

This combination means they are more likely to be self-starters and to make rational and valid choices instead of waiting for approval from others.

It's hard not to judge ourselves, especially when things don't turn out as we planned. The person with a positive self-image is going to reframe the negativity and turn it into something positive.

Live and learn, right? Move forward and make the necessary changes to avoid the same result.

Of course they acknowledge there's a problem, but they know there is also a solution. They are more focused on the solution than allowing defeat to consume and define them. How else can you improve if you don't notice short-comings?

Are You Codependent?

A positive self-image is defined by how you see yourself, not how another sees you. We've covered that much for sure. But sometimes we get caught up in relationships and inadvertently end up placing too much value on how our significant other sees us.

We are ever-changing beings.

We can't expect our partners to always be in love with every single move we make, just like you aren't going to always be elated at their every move. A healthy self-image in a relationship involves nourishing a level of independence that doesn't require constant approval and validation.

Do You Love *You*?

It's the most basic and complicated question there is: Sure, no one is *in love* with every facet of their life. Perhaps we could stand to lose a few pounds or tone that tummy up. Maybe we'd like to feel more confident in a specific area of training. But overall, do you love yourself?

Are you happy with where you are physically, mentally, professionally, financially? And if not, are you actively planning how to remedy those less than desirable qualities? If you answered yes to *any* of those, your self-image is good on this front!

So, what's the verdict? Do you have a positive self-image? Focusing on yourself and taking time for personal growth and development isn't ego, it's you composing a better self-image. A better life.

Engaging in a positive self-image reinforces greater successes in so many areas of your life. Accept yourself, love yourself. It's easier said than done, like mostly everything, but it's worth it. *You* are worth it!

A Positive Attitude at Work Can Boost Your Success

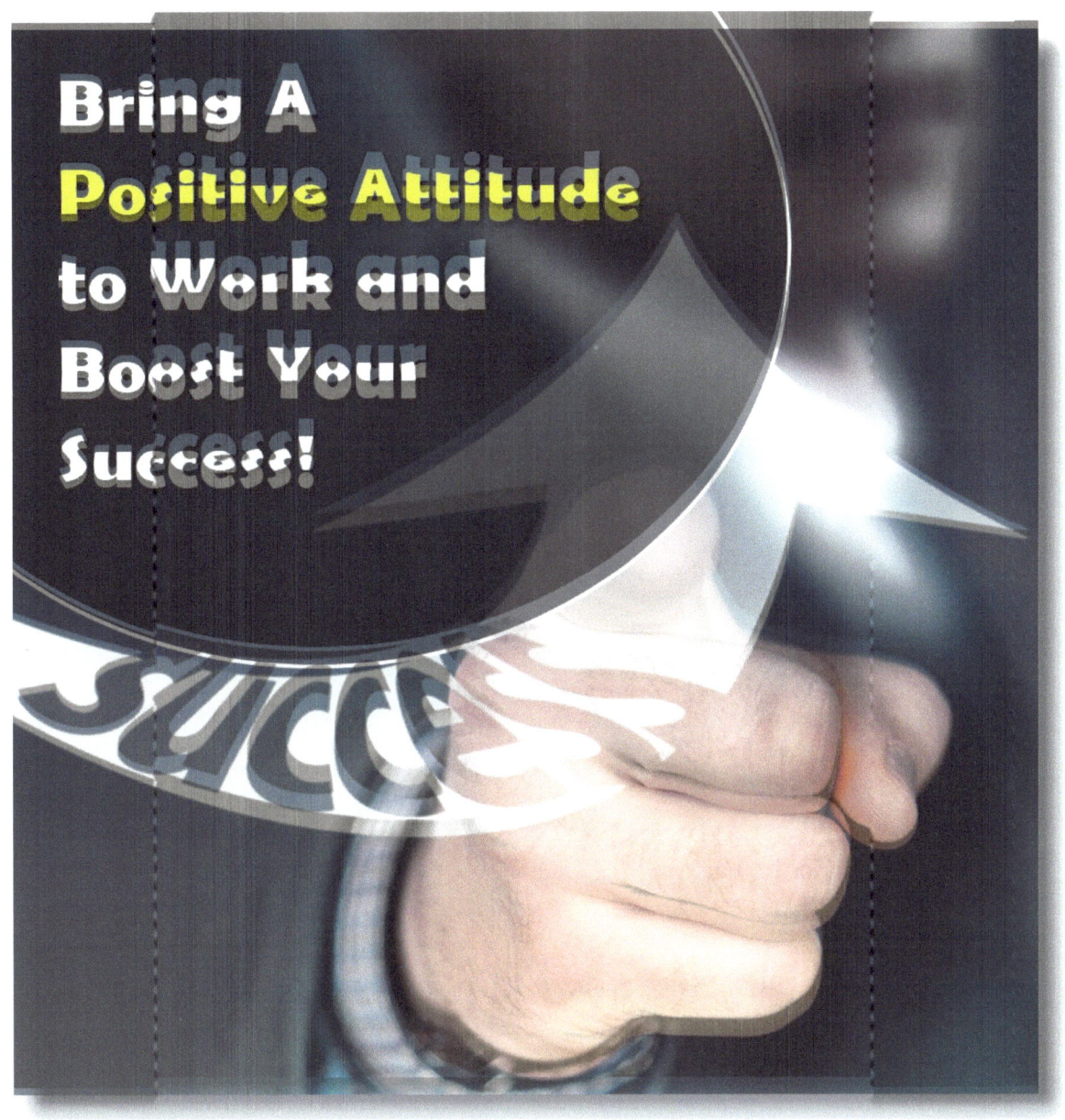

Have you ever seen a car salesman approach you with a frown on his face and complain about the car you're looking to purchase? Of course not! He's got to have a positive attitude to make a sale!

Successful teachers teach with charisma and discipline; they don't spend their time in the classroom whining and kicking their feet. Notable doctors care for their patients with compassion and a knowledge-base to effectively treat them without judgment.

Effective counselors give their clients the tools necessary to get through whatever is troubling them without belittling short-comings.

A positive attitude in the workplace is essential for success!

What To Do – and What Not To Do

Sometimes it can seem impossible to maintain a positive attitude, especially at work. We deal with all sorts of situations and predicaments that aren't always what we hoped for or expected. But if you follow a few simple guidelines, it's easier no matter what comes your way!

Office Gossip is a No-Go

Try to avoid the cliques and hush-hush gossipers. They aren't out for anyone but themselves and will turn on you in a moments' notice. Think about it this way: If they are gossiping *with* you today, they will be gossiping *about* you tomorrow.

Be a Team Player

Get rid of the *me, me, me* attitude and spend your energy working with others to come up with solutions to obstacles. Give credit where credit is due also. There is no "I" in "Team".

Don't Be A Serial Complainer

Nobody needs to be the victim of your foul mood. You stepped in dog poop this morning and it ruined your fancy shoes? Don't take it out on your coworkers. If unusual traffic caused you to be late for a meeting, shake that anguish and disgust off in the parking lot.

Boss riding you for a report that was due last week? When you share your negativity with your peers, you run a great risk of them becoming equally as irritated with *you*.

Keep Your Potty Mouth Shut

If you've got a mouth like a sailor, be sure to keep it shut in the workplace. Even the most innocent of people slip up now and again. Just don't make it a habit.

Speaking with a foul mouth, especially to your superiors, shows an unprofessionalism that might not be overlooked. If you don't have anything nice to say...

Advantages of a Positive Attitude at Work

Why do all of these things?
How can a positive attitude boost your success at work?

You'll Be a Role Model

It could be a seasoned employee or a new-hire, but eventually the superiors are going to come knocking on your cubicle to show someone else the ropes. They will look to *you* to be their shining example of a desirable employee.

Health and Wellness

Stress depletes the immune system. If you are the part of the reason for a stressful environment, think about what that's doing to your body!
With a positive attitude you can help avoid work-related anxieties and better resist any office germs floating around.

Lead Roles

Those with exemplary behavior are often put in lead roles. Instead of being on the phones all day answering calls in the call center, they might just assign you to the lead technician position. Or maybe you'll be chosen to take the lead on an advertising campaign. Whatever the case, it's because of your positive attitude and workplace ethics.

Promotion, Promotion, Promotion!

Let's face it, even the last man or woman on the totem pole is looking to sit in the big chair and have that corner office. Management and the higher ups look for capable beings who meet the criteria for the position, but attitude goes a long, long way. Your positive attitude will have the bosses singing your praise when you're up for a promotion!

Work is sometimes challenging. Deadlines are stressful. It's also hard to constantly maintain a positive attitude when confronted with all of facets of workplace tensions.

Amongst all the stress and strife of the work environment, dealing with many different personalities along with your duties of employment, it takes a great deal of effort to keep a steady flow of positivity.

Keep your head up and stand firm on your ethics. You won't even need to draw attention to your positive attitude; your colleagues and superiors will take notice and reward you in one way or another.

Success is imminent for those who deserve it!

Positive Thinking is Great, Positive 'Action' is Better!

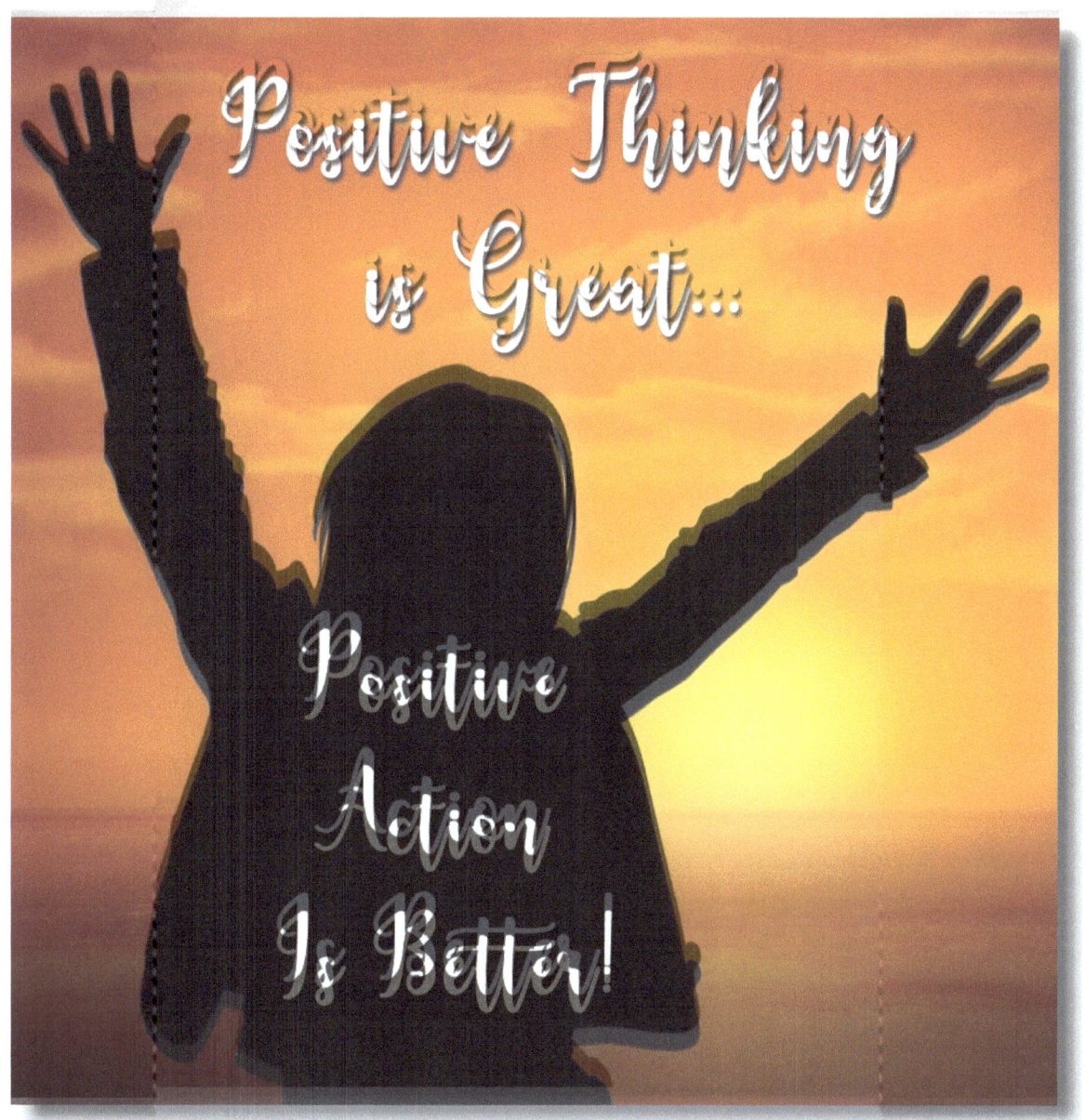

Creating a more meaningful and purposeful life with positive thinking is a great starting place, but very little will truly change without *action*! A vehicle can't go anywhere until it's put in 'drive'. You can devise all sorts of plans and think happy thoughts until the cows come home. Until you take action, nothing moves.

An interesting tidbit: One invokes the other. In fact, one requires the other to be effective. Positive thinking leads to positive action as much as positive action stimulates positive thinking.

Emotion First, Then Behavior

Feeling positive is an emotion, as much as feeling happy or sad. Taking back control of your own positivity and using that as a driving force in your life is excellent. It promotes better health, decreased anxiety and depression, and overall satisfaction with your life and goals.

But having emotion without a follow-up behavior is useless. You are basically standing idle without much progress.
Eventually you'll get discouraged and lose your hold on positive thinking.

Professional Example

Let's say you are going to a board meeting and have to present an idea you think will be a great asset to the company. Sure, you're a little nervous about how receptive the other board members will be, but you have a positive attitude about it.

You have all your ducks in a row; you are completely prepared. You've got an answer for any questions that might show resistance. When you get in there you nail it! Whether they approve of your idea or not, you went in there confident, positive and prepared.

Personal Example

Your significant other is not carrying his weight around the house. Chores are building up and you feel like he's taking advantage of you by not helping out more.

With a positive attitude you approach your spouse and avoid 'blame' words. Surprisingly enough, he's receptive to your new approach and agrees to help take some of the load off you.

Social Example

You run across a non-profit organization that means something to you. You'd like to help out in one way or another, but don't really know where to start. Your positive thinking is the beginning, and only when you put it into action and volunteer do you feel satisfied.

Behavior First, Then Emotion

Going after a positive action first gets the ball rolling in many cases. We don't always *feel* like doing something, but afterward we certainly *feel* better. More positive. More willing to carry out the same action many times over so we can get that positive rush again.

Positive action (moving toward a goal) strengthens positivity and resolve, and requires much less impulsion to keep moving forward.

Professional Example

You notice a coworker is having a rough day. It's affecting other people in the office and causing a less than ideal attitude overall. You make it a point to go by their desk and tell them something you appreciate about them.

It brings a smile to their face and in turn, you feel better. You feel more positive about the day and work environment.

Personal Example

Maybe you're feeling a little down on yourself lately and don't feel very attractive. You stop by the nail salon and get your toes and nails done.

Upon leaving you notice you have boosted self-confidence and positive self-image.

Social Example

Out of nowhere you decide to buy a coffee for the guy behind you. You don't even stay long enough to notice their reaction, but it makes you feel good! A random act of kindness doesn't just enhance the strangers' day, but also your own.

Completing the Circle of Self-motivation

Positive thinking is great, but when you put it into action you receive the true gift and jubilation of a positive life. It doesn't matter which one comes first in the grand scheme of things. We don't always want to go to the gym and workout, but afterward we feel great, right?

It's the action that makes it all come full circle in the realm of positivity. Sure, it takes effort, but what in this world that's truly worth having doesn't take a little elbow grease?

Don't be afraid to put your positive thinking into action. The rewards are life-changing!

Tips to Overcome Negative Thoughts

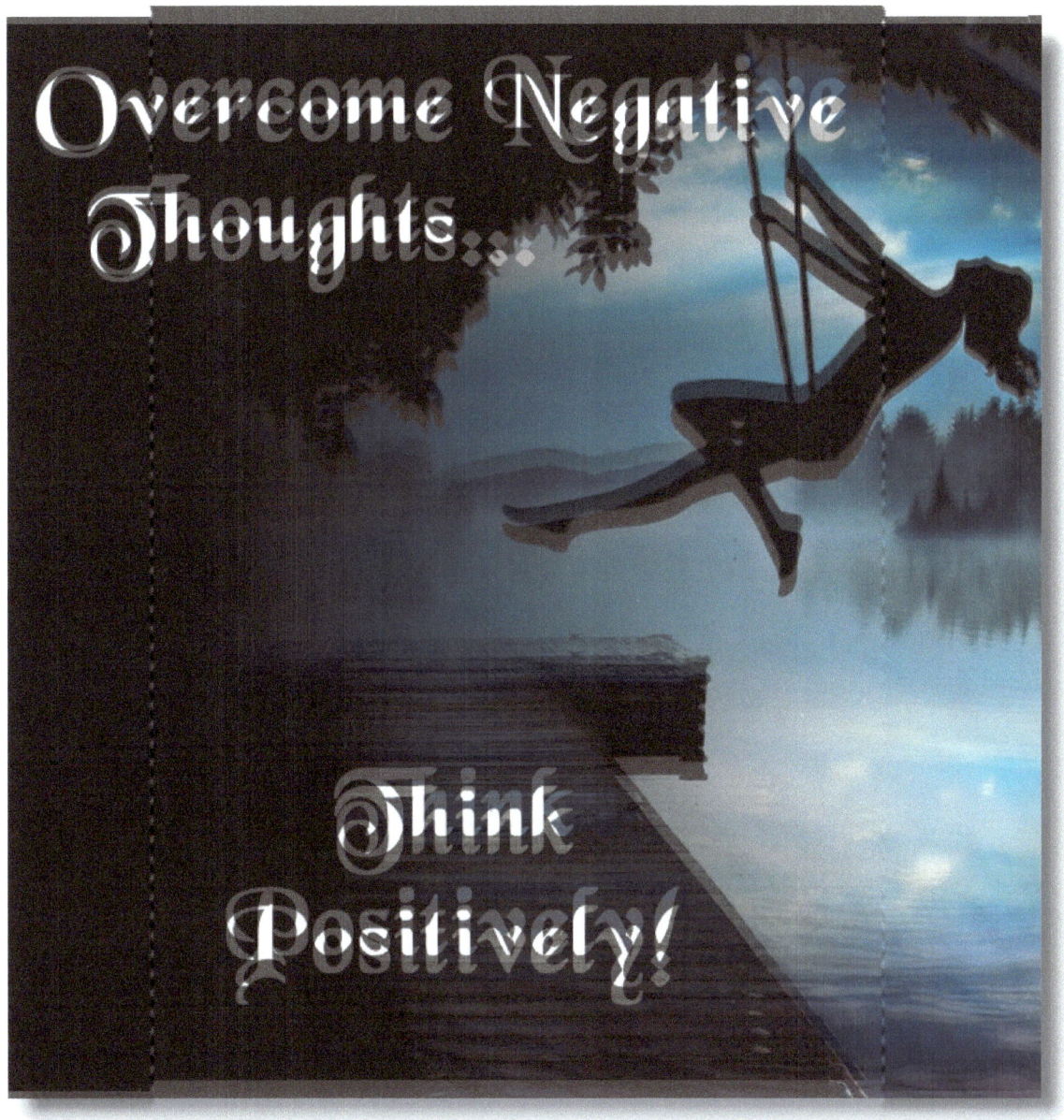

You wouldn't be human if negativity didn't sometimes creep up in your mind and thoughts. As a species we are naturally self-preserving and social creatures with cognitive thinking skills:

If a situation that comes up triggers a fear response, we act accordingly. It's when the negativity consumes us we end up being miserable, and often lonely as a result.

We don't have to be engulfed by negative thoughts. We are all capable of positivity, but we must work at it. Below you'll find tips to overcome your negative thoughts and discover a more meaningful and positive life!

Eggs, Bacon and Positivity!

Wake up and smile. Seriously…. Smile. You have life, breath and a desire to make this the best day ever! From the moment you open your eyes you begin setting the tone for your day. Don't waste these precious minutes! Smile, stretch, and say something good about yourself.

Set realistic goals for the day, remind yourself of the future goals you are aiming for and get your motivation in gear. Some people like to see sticky-notes plastered on their mirrors featuring positivity mantras.

Others enjoy listening to a podcast or radio show. Anything that causes you to laugh, smile and *believe* today is going to be awesome!

Give Negative Surroundings the Boot!

It's important to identify external sources of negativity and get rid of them. Ask yourself, "What are the top 3 things in my life causing negativity?" Be genuine and real with yourself. Once you've identified the sources, brainstorm for positive replacements.

It could be anything from Negative Nancy at work bombarding you with her latest gossip to your kitchen being cluttered and covered with dirty dishes. A lot of us tend to spend entirely too much time on social media and staring at our phones for hours on end, scrolling and scrolling, feeding into the negativity of the world.

Whatever the case, identify it and give it the boot. Tell Negative Nancy you'd rather not be a part of the office dramatics and busy yourself with a good book or window shopping at lunch.

After you do the dishes consider putting a live plant or some fresh cut flowers in the window. Put your phone in a drawer and go work in the garden or go for a walk.

Word Purge!

Writing is a form of therapy for a lot of folks. Some people are verbal processors and talking through it is more effective. If you are feeling particularly anxious or negative about a situation or circumstance, word vomit is a great way to get it out into the universe in a nonjudgmental environment and let it go.

After you've purged all those negative words and feelings, you can really assess the core of the problem and work on a solution.

Q and A Time!

When you feel that negative thought wriggling its way into your mind, you don't have to succumb to the nuisance. Question it. Question the validity of the negativity and give yourself a valid and honest answer.

Is this really something I should take seriously?

Often times there is a co-existing reason for our negative moods and thoughts. Maybe we just got off the phone with an angry customer or our kids are acting like sugar-crazed rascals.

If we stop and question the negative thought at hand, we might find there is another reason for our inability to reason properly and we are making a molehill out of a mountain.

Search and Rescue!

When you find yourself head-on with a legitimately negative force, search for the positive and send out the rescue team to retrieve it. When life hands you lemons... you know the rest. Make a habit of looking for the good. Counteract the negativity with empowering positivity.

Ask yourself questions like:

What can I learn from this?
How would (insert positive friend's name here) handle this situation?
Is there an alternative solution?

Over time, when you make an effort to nip the negativity in the butt, these thoughts become less and less abundant. Pretty soon you won't even be tempted to give negative thoughts the time of day.

They aren't helping you grow, making you happy or paving the way to success. With consistent interruption of the negative thoughts you can create a better you!

Reduce Stress by Reducing Negative Self-Talk

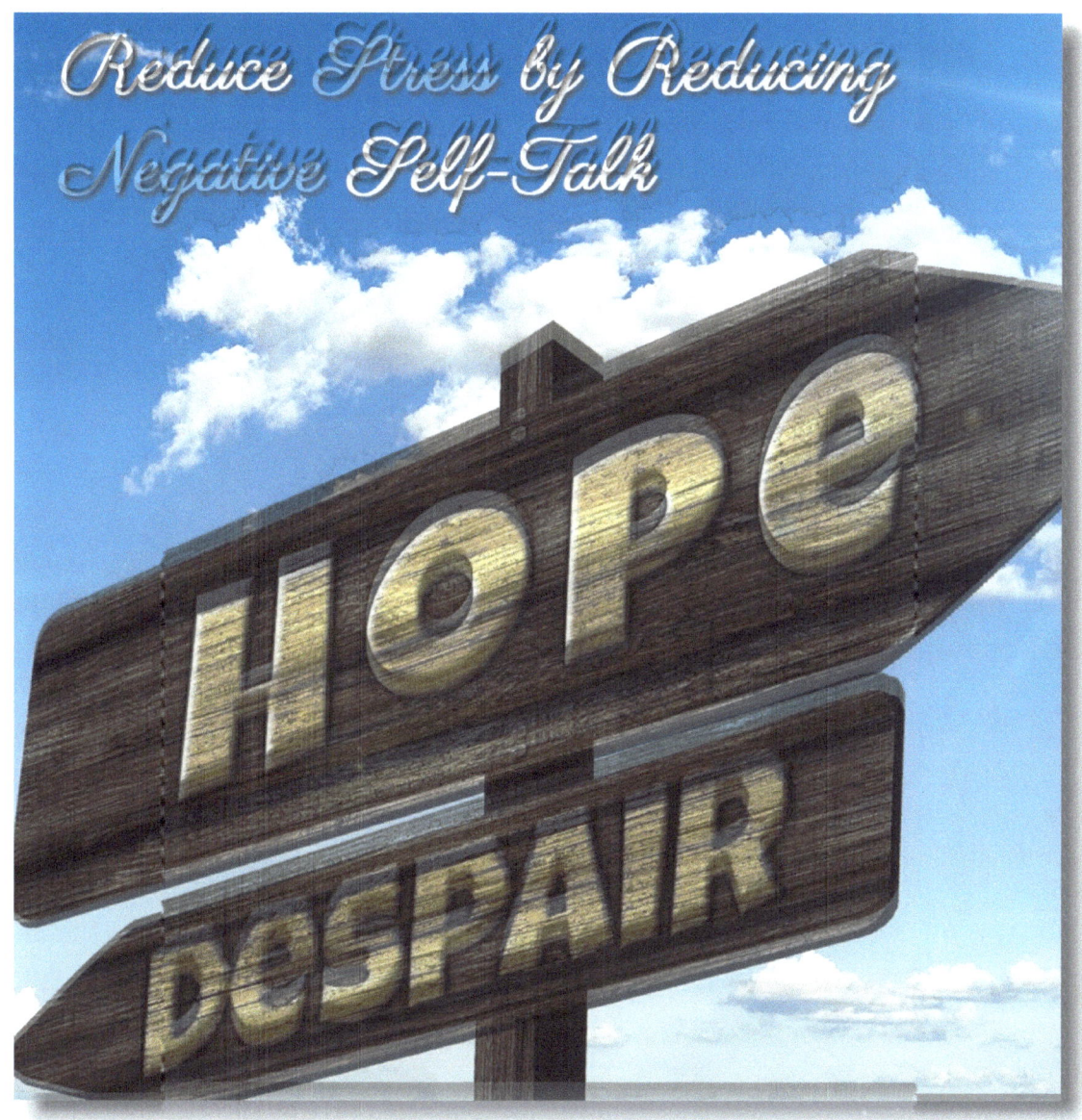

Wouldn't it be nice if we all had our own personal cheering squad constantly feeding us good vibes and encouragement? We would be much less stressed and incredibly confident in our day to day endeavors.

Instead of an entire squad, we can to learn to use our very own inner voices to pull the weight.

Are you your own worst critic? If so, try reducing stress by reducing your negative self-talk.

A little bit of self-criticism goes a long way people, usually too far. You don't have to beat yourself up to get the point across. In fact, engaging in relentless negative self-talk often has the opposite effect.

You will end up regarding yourself as a failure and slide deeper and deeper into the stressful abyss of negativity. Instead, try some of these tips for reducing negative self-talk and in turn, reduce your stress levels.

Permit Imperfections

Have you ever really met a perfect person? They don't exist. Everyone.... let's go over that again... EVERYONE has imperfections. Not a single person on the planet is without dents and dings.

Life throws us all sorts of physical and emotional challenges and we are fools if we believe we can come out unscathed.

It doesn't make you less of a person. It actually makes you well-rounded and capable. You've lived and so far you've survived. Stop telling yourself you are less of a person because you are a survivor with beauty and brawn flowing inside and out!

Shut Up, Negative Nancy!

Give that nasty, negative inner voice a name. When *Rejection Rita* comes bumbling into your thoughts, it's fun to tell her **out loud** to back her truck up and move on down the road.

It might even get a chuckle out of you, because it feels silly calling her out. What you're actually doing is verbally breaking the cycle, the emotional hold, *Pessimistic Paul* how is your stress level at the moment?

Choose Your Words

Words like 'always' and 'never' suggest finality. There's no going back, there's no changing and there's no way out. If you find yourself saying things like, "I never get A's on tests" or "I'm always the slowest to finish," you are setting yourself up for failure.

Why would you try any harder or come up with a solution with such terminal talk?

Erase that negative self-talk and try using less absolute words. For instance you could say, "I may not ace this test, but I'm giving it my all" or "I might be slow, but I finish every time!"

Avoid Assumptions

Not everything is going to go as planned and you can't predict human behavior with absolution. In fact, you only have control of *you* and *your reactions*.

Got stood up for a date?
You haven't received a call for the second interview yet?

Instead of going off the deep end with negative self-talk, maybe there's a logical reason. Don't assume *you* are the reason. Wait for the facts and then process the information. There is no benefit in stressing yourself out over assumptions.

Jot It Down

Journaling is a great tool for noticing patterns in self-talk, as well as allowing your inner voice to be heard and validated. Take a few minutes and write down how you are feeling about the events of the day. Don't put the weight of expectation on what you are writing; just write.

You can physically feel the stress leaving your body as you put it to pen and paper. Now walk away. Come back to your journal entry later and reread it. Are you focused on negative self-talk?

Do you point blame on yourself for things out of your control? And do you feel less emotional and stressed about today than before you wrote it out? It's a verbal purge. When it's out of our heads it's easier to let go.

Promote a Positive Self-Image

If you are spending more time promoting a positive self-image, you have less time to focus on and support a negative self-image. Say good things about yourself. Not just your physical self, but your intellectual, emotional and spiritual sides as well.

Self-image is so much more than outer beauty. Make sure you are balanced and spotlighting all of your incredible qualities. After all, there is only *one* of you!

Reducing negative self-talk takes persistence and patience. It's not something that will happen overnight or even in a week or two. You've got to make a habit of lifting yourself up. Daily stressors today will be reduced and less significant tomorrow if you continue a healthy rule of reducing negative self-talk.

Benefits of Positive Thinking

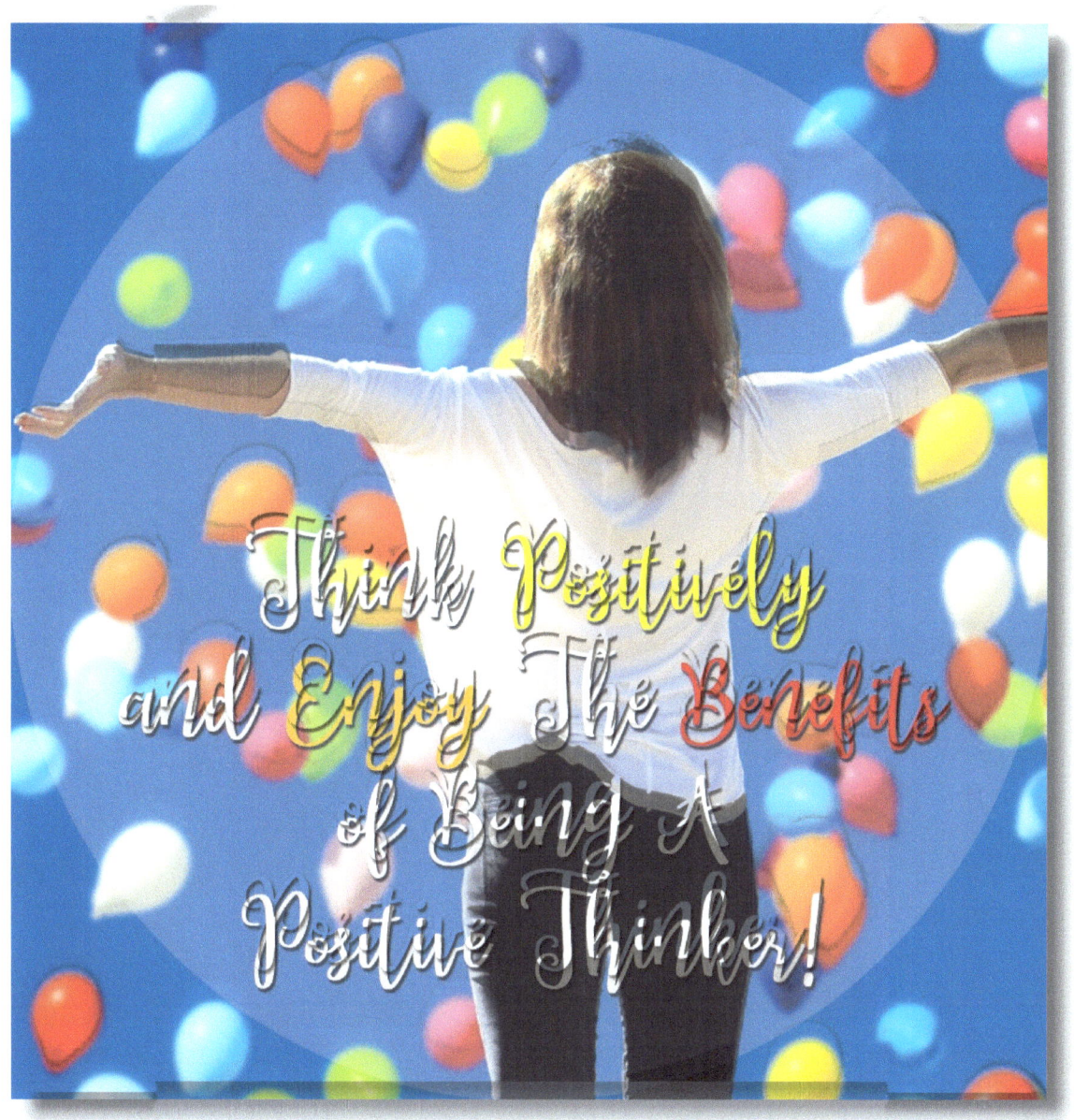

Positive thinking is not just a term; it's a way of life. And it can *change* your life! Life has its twists and turns; there's no doubt about it. Optimism vs pessimism is an internal struggle everyone deals with, especially when we are hit hard with circumstances out of our control.

The benefits of positive thinking overflow into many aspects of our lives and build the foundation for inner peace, happiness and success.

If you never thought a lifestyle of positive thinking could enhance your world, here are a few reasons why you should give it a try:

More Effective Coping Skills

Positive thinkers are better equipped to handle unpleasant situations. Instead of focusing on the negative, positive thinking people spend their energy on solutions. They don't freeze up and stress about a road-block in life. People thinking positively will assess the situation from all sides, weigh it out and figure out how to go around, under or above the wreckage.

A Healthier, Longer Life

Stress and negative thinking affect more than just our self-image and emotions. The physical manifestations of negativity can come in the form of headaches, muscle tension, intestinal problems, depression, anxiety and much more.

Have you ever laid down in bed after a stressful day you felt would never end? Your sleep was probably interrupted multiple times and you just couldn't get your body to relax.

Positive thinkers aren't wound up at the end of the day; they are satisfied with their decisions and know the sun is going to come up tomorrow, just like it did today. This paves the way for a longer, happier life with less health issues.

Appreciate the Good Things

When you are a positive thinker you aren't drowning in self-deprecation and a "why me?" attitude. Instead, you spend more time appreciating even the little things. Very quick to complain, the negative thinker is envious of the next person yet unwilling to seek happiness for himself.

The positive thinker approaches life as a blessing with a multitude of elements delivered in seasons. Maybe this season isn't the best, but you'll make it and be better prepared for next season!

Problems Appear as Opportunities

As you start any day there's no telling what's in store. Any number of situations or circumstances can derail even the most reliable and best-built train. A negative person typically reacts with uncontrolled emotion and gives this setback the power of a full-blown catastrophe of epic proportions. The world is coming to an end and we are all going to die!

The benefit of having a positive attitude allows one to turn this travesty around.

Let go from your job?

Maybe you wanted a career change anyway and now's the perfect time!

Discover your boyfriend cheating?

Now you can plan the singles' cruise you've always wanted to do.

Snowstorm has you homebound?

You've got a stack of romance novels calling your name!

Success

Positive people are picked over negative people time and time again for career advancement. Imagine the two side by side in an interview; who would you pick? With the same educational background and seniority in the company, upper management would be crazy not to choose the positive person.

Would you trust *your* company in the hands of Negative Norman? Sure, he can get the job done but he's going to grunt and complain the whole time. He will bring morale down and cause conflict. The optimistic, positive thinker is not only going to do the job well; he will go above and beyond the call of duty.

He will help his colleagues and be a team player. He might even offer up suggestions on how to build and grow the enterprise.

And that's just career success!

Positive people have more successful interpersonal relationships as well. They choose their words wisely and don't come off as judgmental and hypocritical. Because they aren't out to hurt people or focus on the negative, they are better at effectively communicating with their loved ones.

It's easy to get stuck in a rut and ignore the good. Procuring a habit of positive thinking can transform so many facets of your life. If you want a better life, you have to start somewhere. Given the benefits of positive thinking, it's clearly the better option.

Acknowledgments

This book could not have been completed without the help of many people I hold dear to my heart.

First and foremost, thank you to my dear belated mother and ever present father. From early childhood you taught me to see the inner beauty in each situation and person. You instilled in me the desire to not only persevere but thrive daily in the prodigious moments.

Thank you to my sister. I am in constant awe God allowed me to have a best friend for life. You are unique in so many beautiful ways. I pray you continue using your talents touching the many lives you encounter every day.

Thank you to my extended sisters. I am truly blessed to have you exquisite queens as a source of serenity, adulation and strength. You have held me up when my own crown began to tilt. I thank Abba Father for the many divine pieces each one of you contribute to my life.

Thank you to my friends, family and close ones I love dearly. Your consistent encouragement and inspiration challenge me to pursue new heights daily. Each and every one of you mean so much to me. I love and appreciate the role you play molding my existence.

www.ingramcontent.com/pod-product-compliance
Lightning Source LLC
Chambersburg PA
CBHW051927210526
45473CB00006B/2167